Easy Mediterranean Recipe Book

Quick and Delicious Meals to Boost Your Health

Ben Cooper

Table of Contents

Salmon and Cucumber Salad

Preparation time: 8 minutes
Cooking time: 35 minutes
Servings: 4

Ingredients:

Sauce
1/4 tsp kosher salt
2 tsp lemon juice
13 tsp pepper
1 tbsp olive oil
1 tbsp chopped dill
1 cup yogurt
Cucumber salad
2 tsp olive oil
2 tsp chopped flat-leaf parsley
2 tsp chopped chives
13 tsp pepper
13 tsp kosher salt
1.5 tsp minced shallot
¾ tsp lemon juice
½ lb English cucumbers Salmon and serving
¼ tsp kosher salt
¼ tsp pepper
1 tbsp olive oil Four salmon fillets Dill sprigs

Directions:

1.Mix all the ingredients of the sauce list in a bowl. The sauce is ready.

2.Combine all the items of salad in a bowl and set aside. The salad and dressing are ready.

3.Place fish with skin placed downwards on a baking tray.

4.Grill the fillets for 15 minutes.

5.Place the grilled fillets on a plate and drizzle salad and dressing over it; serve.

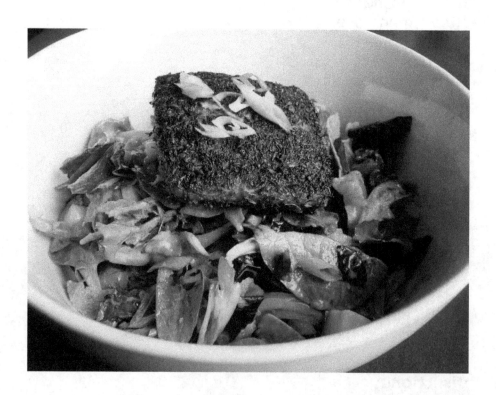

Salmon, Lentil & Pomegranate Salad

Preparation time: 15 minutes
Cooking time: 0 minute
Servings: 2

Ingredients:

1garlic clove chopped
1red onion sliced
1 tsp clear honey
1 pomegranate
140 g hot-smoked salmon
2 tbsp olive oil
2 tbsp chopped tarragon
20 g flat-leaf parsley
400 g lentil juice
½ lemon
toasted pitta bread, to serve

Directions:

1.Combine all the ingredients in a bowl and toss well.

2.Serve and enjoy it.

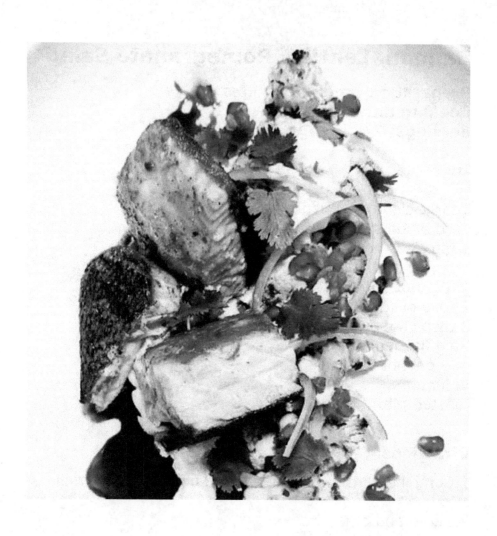

Salmon and pumpkin salad with chili jam

Preparation time: 30 minutes
Cooking time: 30 minutes
Servings: 2

Ingredients:
Lime coriander (chopped to serve)
700 g pumpkin
4salmon fillets
200 g green beans
125 g baby spinach
1 tbsp olive oil
One sliced Spanish onion Dressing
2 tbsp lime juice
1/2 cup vegetable stock (liquid)
1 tbsp fish sauce
1 tbsp chili jam
1 tbsp brown sugar

Directions:

1.Combine all the items of dressing in a pan and boil it for few minutes. The dressing is ready.

2.Drizzle oil over pumpkin and roast in a preheated oven at 200 degrees for 25 minutes.

3.Add peas to boiling water and cook for five minutes.

4.Cook salmon in a heated pan for five minutes.

5.Now mix all the items in a bowl and pour dressing.

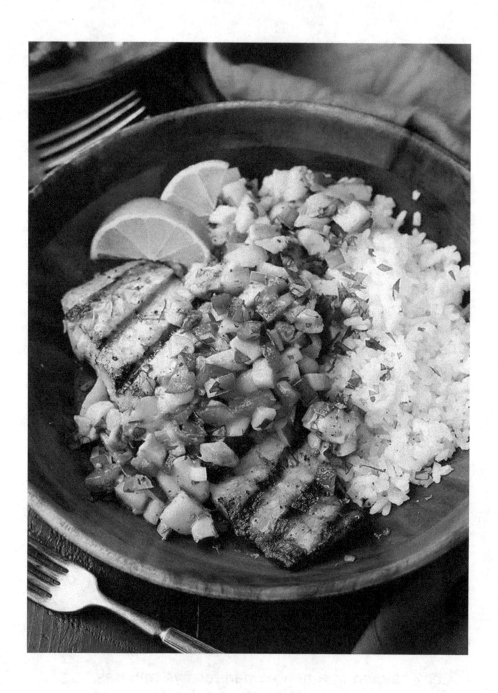

Salmon with Pomegranate Molasses Glaze

Preparation time: 5 minutes
Cooking time: 15 minutes
Servings: 3

Ingredients:

1/2 tsp salt
1/4 cup pomegranate molasses
1/4 tsp cornstarch
2 tsp brown sugar
4 boneless salmon fillets
Black pepper
Pomegranate seeds for garnish
Mint for garnishing

Directions:

1.Whisk pepper, sugar, salt, and starch in a bowl. Coat fillets with the mixture.

2.Fry the fillets in heated oil for five minutes.

3.Transfer the fillets to the baking tray. Drizzle pomegranate molasses over fillets.

4.Bake in a preheated oven at 400 degrees for 15 minutes.

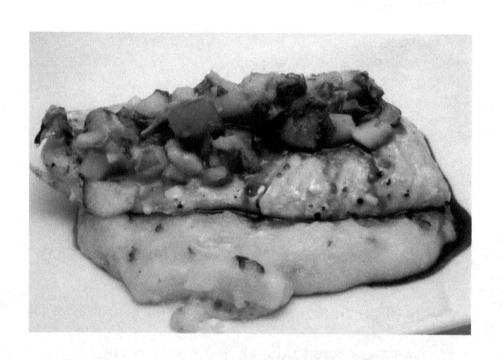

Scallops and Summer Vegetable Skillet

Preparation time: 15 minutes
Cooking time: 15 minutes
Servings: Adjustable

Ingredients:

1/2 cup diced zucchini
1 cup corn kernels
1 sliced cherry tomatoes
1 lb scallops
1 tbsp olive oil
3 cloves garlic minced
3 tbsp diced shallots
3 tbsp salted butter
Salt to taste pepper to taste

Directions:

1.Cook scallops in a heated oven over medium flame for three minutes. Transfer it to a plate.

2.Sauté shallots and garlic in the same pan over medium flame. Stir in zucchini and tomatoes for ten minutes.

3.Mix in corn, salt, and black pepper. Add scallop and cook for five minutes.

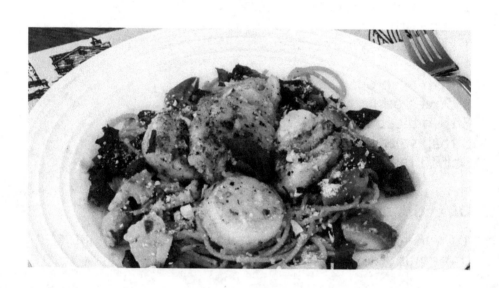

Tuna Patties

Preparation time: 15 minutes
Cooking time: 10 minutes
Servings: 4

Ingredients:

3 tbsp vegetable oil
3 tbsp grated Parmesan cheese
3 tbsp diced Onion
15 oz tuna
2 tsp lemon juice
2 eggs
10 tbsp bread crumbs
1 pinch of black pepper

Directions:

1.Whisk all the items in a bowl.

2.Make patties out of the mixture.

3.Fry the patties in heated oil over medium flame for five minutes.

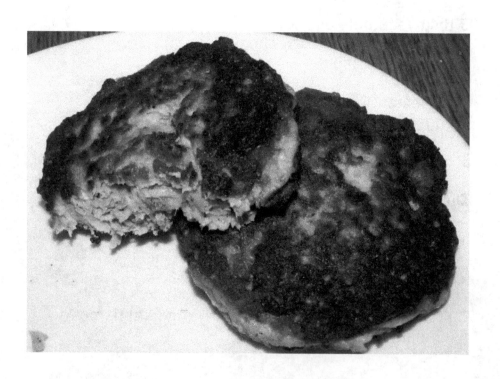

Whole Salmon Fillet with Crispy Lemon & Basil Crumb Topping

Preparation time: 15 minutes
Cooking time: 18 minutes
Servings: 4

Ingredients:

Salt to taste
Black pepper to taste
2 cloves garlic
1.45 lb salmon fillet
1 tbsp lemon juice
1 tbsp lemon thyme
1 lb asparagus
1 lemon, zested
1 cup bread crumbs
½ tsp salt
½ tsp black pepper
1/3 cup grated Parmesan cheese
1/3 cup chopped fresh basil
¼ cup olive oil, divided

Directions:

1.Season salmon with oil, pepper, and salt.

2.Shift the salmon in the pan.

3.Mix asparagus with oil and salt and place around salmon.

4.Blend garlic, cheese, basil, thyme, lemon juice, zest, salt, and pepper in a food processor.

5.Pour the mixture over salmon.

6.Bake in the oven for 20 minutes.

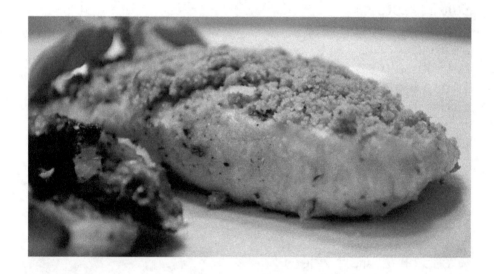

Seafood paella

Preparation time: 15 minutes
Cooking time: 55 minutes
Servings: 6

Ingredients:

2 ¼ cups chicken broth
2 tsp olive oil
1 lb jumbo shrimp
½ teaspoon saffron threads
Salt to taste
8 oz sliced chorizo sausage
2 cloves garlic, minced
1 1/3 cups Arborio rice
1 tsp paprika
1 tbsp olive oil
1 sliced red bell pepper
1 pinch of cayenne pepper
½ yellow onion, diced
½ cup green peas

Directions:

1.Fry chorizo in heated oil for three minutes.

2.Mix in onions and cook for three more minutes.

3.Stir in rice and peas and toss well.

4.Place shrimp over rice and bake for twenty minutes.

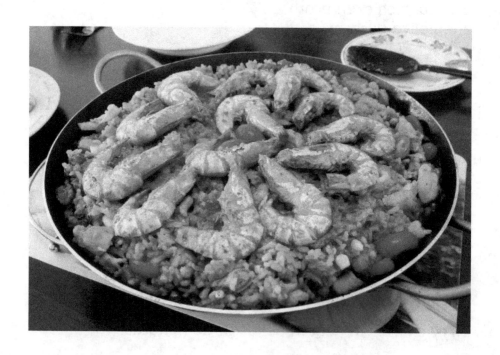

Thyme-Scented Salmon with White Bean Salad

Preparation time: 15 minutes
Cooking time: 0 minute
Servings: 4

Ingredients:
Bean Salad
3 tbsp lemon juice
2 tsp chopped parsley
2 tsp chopped mint
2 tsp chopped basil
2 tbsp water
2 garlic cloves, minced
1 tbsp olive oil
15 oz cannellini beans
½ cup chopped shallots
½ cup chopped carrot
1/3 cup chopped celery
Salmon
Four salmon fillets
3 tbsp lemon juice
2 tsp chopped thyme
13 tsp black pepper
1 tsp chopped parsley
½ tsp salt

Directions:

1.Cook celery, carrot, shallots, and garlic in heated oil over medium flame for five minutes.

2.Mix all the ingredients and cook.

3.Place the mixture in salmon.

4.Bake salmon in a preheated oven at 375 degrees for 15 minutes.

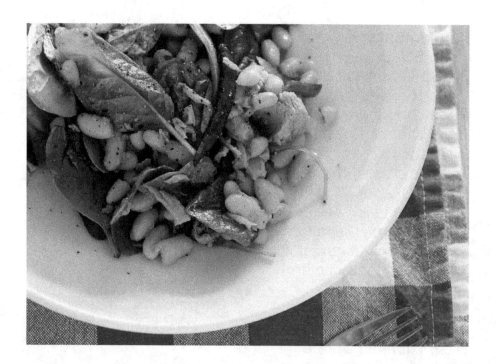

Curry Chicken Salad

Preparation time: 15 minutes
Cooking time: 15 minutes
Servings: 6

Ingredients:

3 cooked chicken breasts
2/3 cup chopped celery
2 tbsp lemon juice
1/4 tsp black pepper
1/4 cup sliced chives
1/3 cup raisins
1/2 tsp salt
1/2 cup roasted salted cashews
1/2 cup mayonnaise
1 tbsp yellow curry powder
1 tart apple

Directions:

1.Whisk all the items in the bowl and serve.

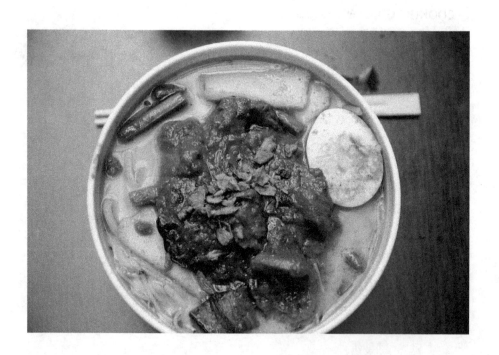

Grilled Indian Chicken

Preparation time: 35 minutes
Cooking time: 10 minutes
Servings: 4

Ingredients:

4 boneless chicken breasts marinade
1/4 tsp cayenne pepper
1/2 tsp ginger
1/2 cup plain yogurt
1 tsp cumin
1 tsp coriander
1 tbsp paprika
1 tbsp onion powder
1 tbsp minced garlic
1 tbsp lemon juice
1 tbsp garam masala
1 tbsp cilantro leaves

Directions:

1.Combine all the items in a bowl and set aside.

2.Grill chicken over a grill for seven minutes from both sides.

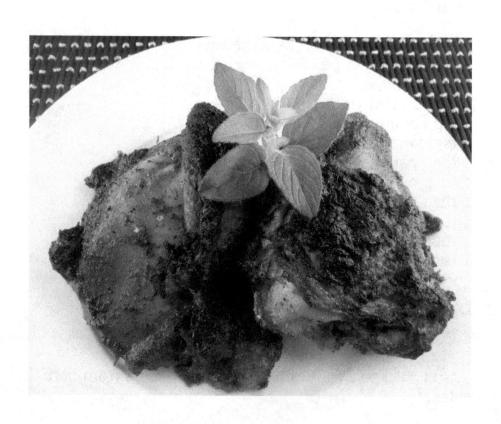

Hearty Turkey Stew

Preparation time: 10 minutes
Cooking time: 60 minutes
Servings: 4

Ingredients:

100 g sliced bacon lardons
1/3 cup heavy cream
1 tbsp butter
1 leek
2 sliced
Carrots Two stalks celery diced
2 cloves garlic pressed
2 tbsp flour, heaped
4 cups chicken or turkey stock
2 cups cooked turkey
2 chopped potatoes
2 bay leaves
1 tbsp thyme leaves
1 tbsp chopped parsley
salt e pepper to taste

Directions:

1.Fry bacon in butter over medium flame. Stir in leeks, carrots, thyme, and celery, and cook for five minutes. Mix garlic and cook again for one minute.

2.Add flour, pepper, and salt.

3.Mix potatoes, bay leaves, and turkey and cook for 50 minutes.

4.Add heavy cream and serve.

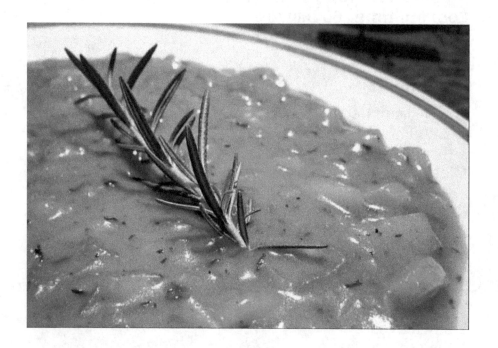

Herb and Orange Chicken

Preparation time: 10 minutes
Cooking time: 60 minutes
Servings: 4

Ingredients:

1/4 cup ghee
3 1/2 oranges
4.5 lb chicken
3 yellow potatoes
2 stems of rosemary
6 stems of thyme
Salt & pepper

Directions:

1.Heat orange juice in ghee over medium flame and set aside.

2.Place chicken, potatoes, orange slices, thyme, and rosemary.

3.Bake for one hour and serve with orange sauce.

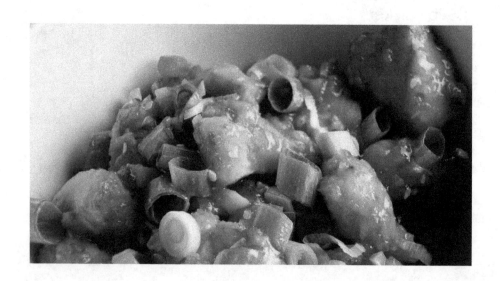

Pomegranate Walnut & Chicken Stew

Preparation time: 15 minutes
Cooking time: 75 minutes
Servings: 5

Ingredients:
1 cups California walnuts
Pinch salt & pepper
2 tbsp olive oil
1 tbsp butter
4 cloves garlic chopped
1 tsp turmeric
1 tsp cumin
1 cinnamon stick
½ tsp nutmeg
½ tsp black pepper orange zest
2 cups chicken stock
2 tbsp maple
1 ½ tsp salt One chickpea
Serve with Persian Rice
Garnish using chopped Italian parsley Garnish with pomegranate seeds
1–1 ½ lb chicken thighs
3 cups yellow onion, diced
1/4 cup pomegranate molasses

Directions:

1.Roast the walnuts over medium flame.

2.Blend the roasted walnuts.

3.Cook chicken in a Dutch oven in heated oil. Set aside.

4.Fry onions in heated oil for five minutes.

5.Stir in garlic and sauté for five minutes.

6.Mix cinnamon, nutmeg, cumin, zest, and turmeric and sauté for a minute.

7.Pour in stock, chicken, syrup, molasses, walnuts, salt, and simmer for 45 minutes.

8.Add the chickpeas and boil it for 15 minutes.

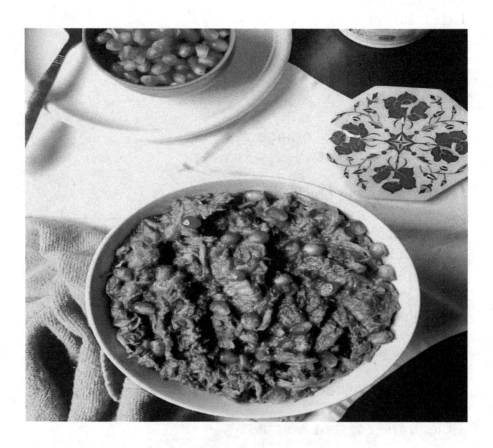

Roasted Chicken and White Bean Medley

Preparation time: 20 minutes
Cooking time: 60 minutes
Servings: 4

Ingredients:

8 teaspoons Dijon mustard
8 skin-on bone-in chicken thighs (about 2 pounds)
2 tablespoons olive oil
2 tablespoons coarsely chopped fresh parsley
2 tablespoons capers with brine
2 (15-ounce) cans white beans, drained and rinsed
1/2 teaspoon freshly ground black pepper
1 large lemon, thinly sliced, seeds removed
1 1/2 teaspoons kosher salt

Directions:

1.Preheat oven to 425 °F.

2.In a baking dish, toss capers, beans & distribute them
on the tray.
3.Spread mustard in beans & capers on the skin of
every chicken. Put lemon pieces all around & beneath
chicken & add insufficient water.

4.Spice the dish with black pepper & sea salt & spray
chicken with oil.

5.Insert the instant-read thermometer in chicken and
roast it until skin becomes brown for thirty-five minutes

6.Switch the pan on the lower rack of the oven if the chicken starts to smoke while finishing the frying process.

7.Place prepared chicken in a bowl and decorate it with slices of lemon, capers, & beans. Put chicken sauce across the bowl and sprinkle it with parsley.

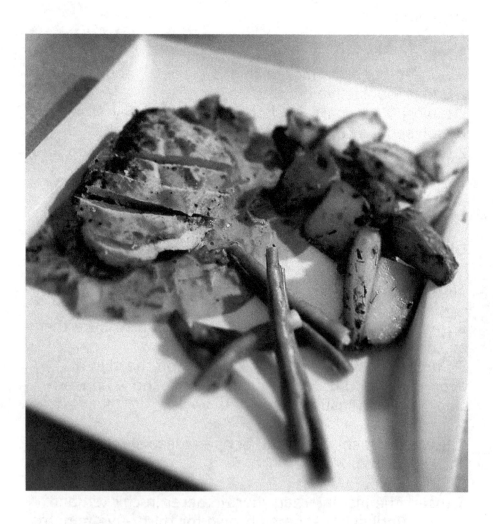

South-Western Chicken Salad

Preparation time: 10 minutes
Cooking time: 0 minutes
Servings: 6

Ingredients:

1 cup crushed tortilla chips
1 and 1/2 cups black beans
1 and 1/2 cups corn
1 avocado, diced
1 teaspoon minced garlic
1/2 cup plain Greek yogurt (use nonfat)
1/2 jalapeño, finely diced
1/2 red onion, diced
1 teaspoons apple cider vinegar
2 heaping teaspoons taco seasoning (use mild)
2 teaspoons honey
2 tomatoes, diced
3 Tablespoons extra virgin olive oil
3/4 cup shredded cheddar cheese
6 cups chopped romaine lettuce
6 cups cubed cooked chicken*
Dressing handful chopped cilantro juice of 1 lime
Salt, to taste and if needed

Directions:

1.Add all the ingredients to the bowl and mix them except salt

2.Pour the dressing over the salad and toss it.

3.Serve it cold.

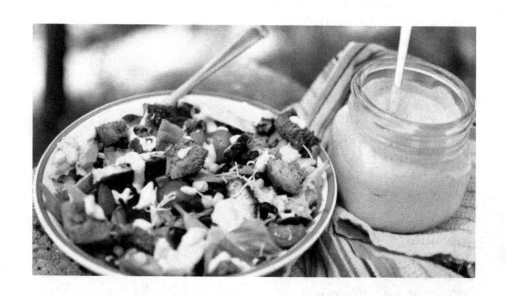

The best turkey chili ever

Preparation time: 15 minutes
Cooking time: 60 minutes
Servings: 1

Ingredients:

3 cloves of garlic, minced
2 teaspoons hot sauce
2 tablespoons olive oil
2 tablespoons chili powder
2 pounds lean ground turkey
2 cups chicken or vegetable broth
1/2 teaspoon cayenne pepper (optional)
1 yellow pepper, chopped
yellow bell pepper, chopped
1 teaspoon garlic powder
1 teaspoon dried oregano
1 teaspoon dried basil
1 tablespoon brown sugar
1 sweet onion, finely chopped
1 red bell pepper, chopped
1/2 teaspoon sea salt
28oz crushed tomatoes
28oz black beans, drained
15oz petite diced tomatoes
15oz of kidney or pinto beans
Toppings: Sour cream, green onions, limes, shredded
cheddar cheese

Directions:

1.Heat the olive oil in a heavy bottom pot over medium-
high & heat it till it shimmers.

2.Add-In the ground turkey & simmer for 9 minutes, smashing it individually with a wooden spoon's help until it turned brown.

3.Add more olive oil if needed & whisk in onions & garlic.

4.Cook for 3 minutes before soften & fragrant.

5.Add peppers & again cook for three more minutes.

6.Place the fried turkey in the pot again & then add the remaining ingredients to it.

7.Stir & bring to a boil once combined.

8.Simmer this till the chili cooked completely 7 left it uncovered for 45 to 65 minutes until it becomes dense

Warm Chicken Pasta Salad

Preparation time: 5 minutes

Cooking time: 18 minutes

Servings: 3

Ingredients:

375g dried rigatoni pasta

500g Lilydale Free Range Chicken Breast, trimmed

One medium brown onion, thinly sliced

One garlic clove, crushed

200g semi-dried tomatoes, drained, chopped

300ml pure cream

50g baby rocket

1/2 teaspoon dried chili flakes 1/4 cup olive oil

Directions:

1.Take frypan and cook pasta until it becomes soft to follow the pasta packet's instructions and drain the remaining water.

2.Along with that, heat 1 tbsp. Oil in a pan and add chicken to it.

3.Cook every side until it is completely cooked. Remove frypan from the stove, cover it & set it aside for 6 minutes.

4.Take the remaining oil in a frypan, heat it over medium heat, and then add the onion. Cook for 4 to 6 minutes, mix frequently, or till the onion has softened.

5.Onions, Garlic, & chili are added. Cook for 1 minute or till the smell is floral.

6.Now add cream, then cook for 4 to 6 minutes, or till the mixture thickens, stirring regularly.

7.Put a bowl of spaghetti, chicken, and rocket. Add the onions mixture. To combine, toss. Just serve.

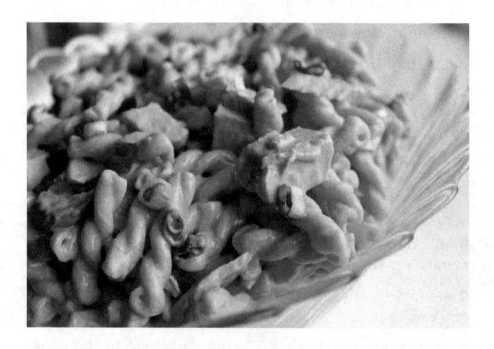

Cinnamon Buckwheat Bowls

Preparation Time: 5 minutes

Cooking Time: 15 minutes

Servings: 1

Ingredients:

½ cup buckwheat groats, rinsed

½ cup almond milk or milk of choice

½ teaspoon cinnamon

½ cup water

½ teaspoon vanilla Honey to serve Sliced fruit to serve

Directions:

1.In a small saucepan, add washed buckwheat grains, water, almond milk, cinnamon, and vanilla. Boil and then simmer and cover with a lid. Cook over low heat for 10 minutes.

2.Turn off the heat and steam, covered, for an additional 5 minutes.

3.Pour with a fork and divide it into a bowl. Fill with fruit slices, sprinkle more milk and chopped honey if desired.

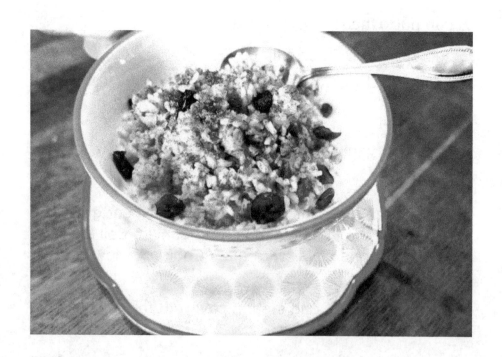

Arugula, Egg, and Charred Asparagus Salad

Preparation Time: 5 minutes

Cooking Time: 15 minutes

Servings: 4

Ingredients:

oz. medium asparagus, trimmed

½ teaspoon black pepper, divided large eggs in shells

1 tablespoon fresh lemon juice

oz. baby arugula

1 tablespoon extra-virgin olive oil

1 tablespoon water

¼ cup plain whole-milk Greek yogurt

1 teaspoon kosher salt, divided

Directions:

1.Preheat broiler to high.

2.Bring a small saucepan filled with water to a boil. Carefully add eggs. Cook for 8 minutes.

3.Place eggs in a bowl filled with ice water and let stand for 2 minutes. Peel eggs, cut into quarters and sprinkle with ¼ teaspoon salt and 1/8 teaspoon pepper.

4.Combine olive oil, ¼ teaspoon salt, ¼ teaspoon pepper, and asparagus on a baking sheet. Spread in a single layer in pan. Boil for 3 minutes or until lightly

45

charred. Remove asparagus mixture from the pan and cut into 2 inch pieces.

5.Combine remaining ¼ teaspoon salt, remaining 1/8 teaspoon pepper, yogurt, juice, and 1 tablespoon water in a medium bowl, stirring with a whisk. Add arugula and toss.

6.Arrange arugula mixture on a platter. Top with asparagus mixture and eggs. Enjoy!

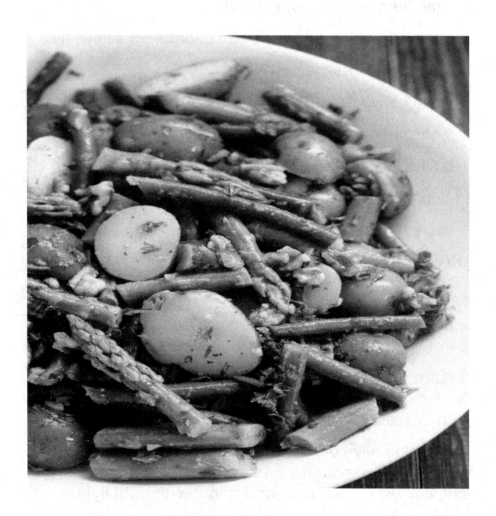

Spring Vegetable and Quinoa Salad with Bacon

Preparation Time: 5 minutes

Cooking Time: 10 minutes

Servings: 4

Ingredients:

1 ¾ cups ginger-coconut quinoa

1 cups fresh asparagus, cut diagonally into 1 inch pieces center-cut bacon slices, chopped

1 tablespoon unsalted butter tablespoons cider vinegar

½ cup frozen green peas

1 teaspoons whole-grain Dijon mustard

oz. baby spinach

tablespoons sliced almonds, toasted

1 teaspoon black pepper

1 tablespoon fresh thyme leaves

1 tablespoon chopped fresh tarragon

½ cup chopped fresh flat-leaf parsley

Directions:

1.Boil a large pot filled with water. Add asparagus and peas. Boil for 2 minutes, then drain. Plunge into a bowl of ice water and drain.

2.Cook the bacon in a large saucepan over medium-high heat, stirring occasionally. Remove bacon from the pan with a slotted spoon. Set aside.

3.Add vinegar, butter, and Dijon mustard to drippings in the pan, stirring with a whisk until butter melts. Add quinoa and pepper to the pan—cook for 1 minute.

4.Place quinoa mixture in a medium bowl. Add asparagus mixture, parsley, tarragon, thyme, and spinach, tossing to combine. Divide quinoa mixture among 4 plates; sprinkle evenly with reserved bacon and almonds.

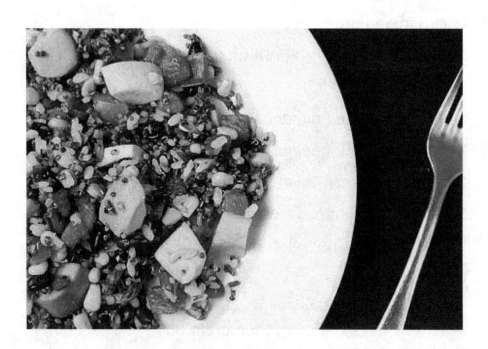

Golden Chicory in Prosciutto Wraps

Preparation Time: 20 minutes

Cooking Time: 55 minutes

Servings: 1

Ingredients:

1 heads of chicory

Slices prosciutto or Serrano ham

75 ml vegetable stock or white wine

1 tablespoons butter

1 tablespoons Dijon mustard

¼ cup whipping cream thyme sprigs slices, about 2 oz. melting cheese (cheddar is great) Sauté potatoes and green salad to serve

Directions:

1.Preheat oven to 350 °F. Cut a cross from the base in the middle of the end of each chicory head.

2.Fill the butter in the grooves, and then place the slices of Serrano ham in pairs on the work surface, overlapping them slightly.

3.Paint the ham with mustard and spread the radish on top. Pull each radish head away from you, comfortably wrapping it in the ham.

4.Place the radish wrapped in an oven or small skillet, pour over the vegetable stock or white wine on top with the thyme sprigs. Cover the plate with loose foil and bake for 30-40 minutes until the radish is soft.

5.Unlock the plate, place the cheese slices on the chicory and bake, keep uncovered for another 6-8 minutes, until the cheese is melted and browned. The radish is now ready to serve.

6.For an extra touch, remove the chicory, place the pan on medium heat and boil the juices with the cream for 4-5 minutes until they are rich and syrupy.

7.Pour the sauce over the radish. Serve with sautéed potatoes and salad.

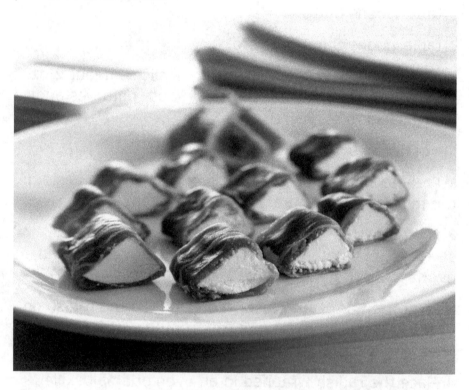

Vegetable Cabbage Soup

Preparation Time: 5 minutes

Cooking Time: 15 minutes

Servings: 6

Ingredients:

½ large head cabbage, chopped

1 large onion, chopped

stalks celery, minced carrots, chopped

tablespoons extra virgin olive oil cloves garlic, minced

½ teaspoon chili powder

1 can white beans, draineed and rinsed

1 can chopped fire-roasted tomatoes 1 pinch red pepper flakes

1 teaspoon thyme leaves

1 cups low-sodium vegetable broth

1 tablespoons freshly of chopped parsley, and more for garnish Kosher salt

Freshly ground black pepper cups water

Directions:

1.In a large pot over medium heat, heat olive oil. Add onion, celery, and carrots, and season with salt, pepper, and chili powder.

2.Cook, stirring often, until vegetables are soft, 5 to 6 minutes. Stir in beans, thyme, and garlic and cook until garlic is fragrant, about 30 seconds. Add broth and water, and bring to a simmer.

3.Stir in tomatoes and cabbage and simmer until cabbage is wilted, about 6 minutes.

4.Remove from heat and stir in red pepper flakes, and parsley. Season to taste with salt and pepper. Garnish with more parsley, if desired. Enjoy!

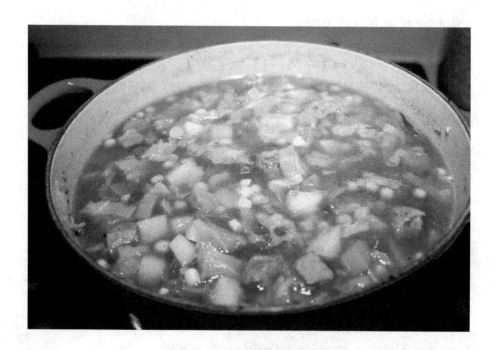

Fresh Herb Frittata

Preparation Time: 10 minutes

Cooking Time: 15 minutes

Servings: 6

Ingredients:

2 fresh eggs

1 tablespoons chopped fresh parsley

1 tablespoons chopped fresh oregano

1 scallions, sliced thin, using both white and green parts

½ cup heavy cream

¾ cup finely grated parmesan cheese, divided into ½ cup and 1/4 cup portions

Salt and pepper to taste

Directions:

1.Preheat oven to 400 °F.

2.In a medium mixing bowl, combine eggs, parsley, scallions, oregano,½ cup of cheese, and heavy cream.

3.Whisk together until thoroughly combined—season with salt and pepper, to taste.

4.In a 10-inch spicy cast iron pot, heat about 1 tablespoon of olive oil over medium heat.

5.Add the egg mixture and cook for about 5 minutes or until the edges start to come out.

6.Sprinkle the remaining cup of cheese over the eggs.

7.Transfer the skillet to the oven and bake for 10-12 minutes, or until the cakes are puffy, the edges are visible and shake a little in the center.

8.Bake on low for about 30-45 seconds to brown the lid.

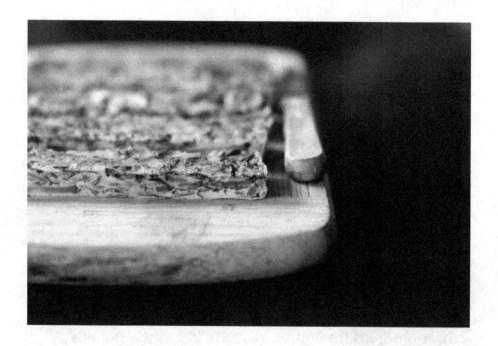

Herb-Roasted Olives and Tomatoes

Preparation Time: 10 minutes

Cooking Time: 20 minutes

Servings: 4

Ingredients:

1 cup Greek olives

1 cup garlic-stuffed olives cups cherry tomatoes

1 cup pitted ripe olives

1 tablespoon herbs de Provence tablespoons olive oil

garlic cloves, peeled

¼ teaspoon pepper

Directions:

1.Preheat oven to 425 °F.

2.Combine cherry tomatoes, garlic-stuffed olives, Greek olives, pitted ripe olives, and garlic cloves on a greased baking pan.

3.Add oil and seasonings. Toss to coat. Roast until tomatoes are softened, 15-20 minutes, stirring occasionally.

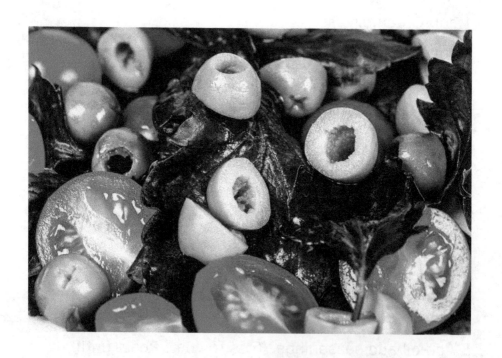

Grilled Asparagus with Caper Vinaigrette

Preparation Time: 5 minutes

Cooking Time: 10 minutes

Servings: 6

Ingredients:

1 ½ pounds asparagus spears, trimmed teaspoons caper, coarsely chopped

1 tablespoon red wine vinegar

1 garlic clove, minced

1 tablespoons extra virgin olive oil

¼ cup small basil leaves

½ teaspoon Dijon mustard Cooking spray

½ teaspoon kosher salt, divided

¼ teaspoon freshly ground black pepper

Directions:

1.Preheat grill to medium-high heat.

2.Place asparagus in a shallow dish. Add 1 tablespoon oil and ¼ teaspoon salt, tossing well to coat.

3.Place asparagus on grill rack coated with cooking spray.

4.Grill 4 minutes or until crisp-tender, turning after 2 minutes.

5.Combine remaining ¼ teaspoon salt, vinegar, mustard, and garlic.

6.Stir with a whisk. Slowly pour remaining 2 tablespoons oil into vinegar mixture, stirring constantly with a whisk. Stir in capers.

7.Arrange asparagus on a serving platter. Drizzle with vinaigrette, and sprinkle with basil.

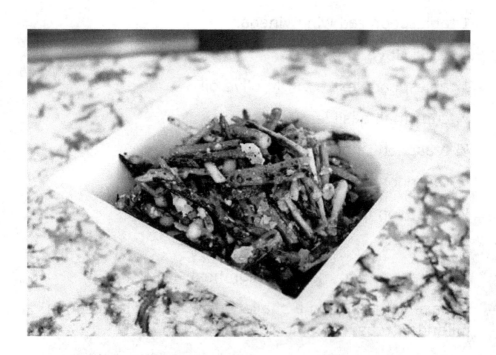

Herby Pork with Apple & Chicory Salad

Preparation Time: 5 minutes

Cooking Time: 15 minutes

Servings: 4

Ingredients:

oz. pork tenderloin, trimmed of any sinew and fat large apples, cored and sliced

270g pack chicory, leaves separated

1 tablespoon honey

1 tablespoon walnut oil

1 tablespoon chopped parsley

1 tablespoon chopped tarragon teaspoons wholegrain mustard Juice of 1 lemon

Directions:

1.Preheat oven to 350°F. Grate pork with 1 teaspoon oil, 1 teaspoon mustard, and a few spices.

2.Brown, transfer to a baking sheet and squeeze half of the herbs. Bake for 15 minutes until well cooked.

3To make the salad, mix the lemon juice, honey, and the rest of the walnut oil and mustard.

4.Period and add apples, radishes, and other herbs. Serve the sliced pork with the salad on the side.

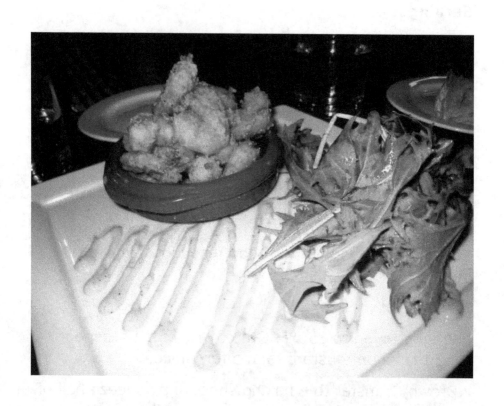

Tomato Green Bean Soup

Preparation Time: 15 minutes

Cooking Time: 30 minutes

Servings: 4

Ingredients:

1 ½ cups diced fresh tomatoes

½ cup chopped onion

½ pound fresh green beans cut into

1 inch pieces

½ cup chopped carrots

1/8 cup minced fresh basil

½ garlic clove, minced

¼ teaspoon salt

1/8 teaspoon pepper

1 teaspoon butter

cups reduced-sodium vegetable broth

Directions:

1.In a large saucepan, sauté onion and carrots in butter for 5 minutes.

2.Stir in the broth, green beans and garlic. Bring to a boil. Reduce heat.

3.Cover and simmer until vegetables are tender.

4.Stir in the tomatoes, basil, salt and pepper. Cover and simmer 5 minutes longer.

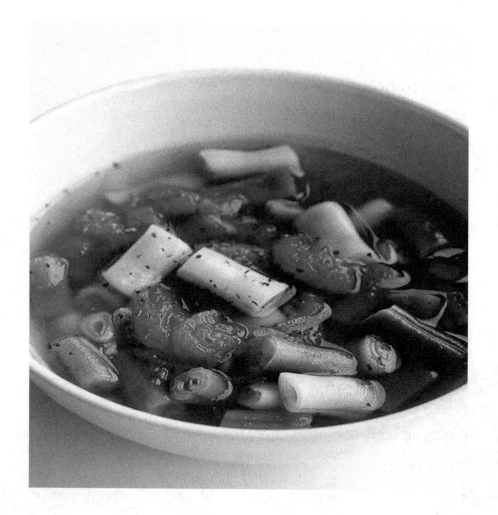

Kale Salad with Pecorino and Lemon

Preparation Time: 5 minutes

Cooking Time: 0 minutes

Servings: 4

Ingredients:

1 large bunch kale, washed and trimmed of steams lemons, juiced

1 ounces Pecorino Romano, grated

½ cup olive oil

Kosher salt and fresh black pepper to taste

Directions:

1.Wrap several cabbage leaves lengthwise and cut off the thick central stem using the tip of a knife. On the other hand, wrap the remaining pile of dehydrated leaves in a tight cigar shape and cut them into thin ribbons.

2.Discard the grated cabbage with the cheese. Lightly beat the lemon juice and olive oil and pour over the salad.

3.Try and season with salt and pepper. Let the salad sit at room temperature for an hour before serving.

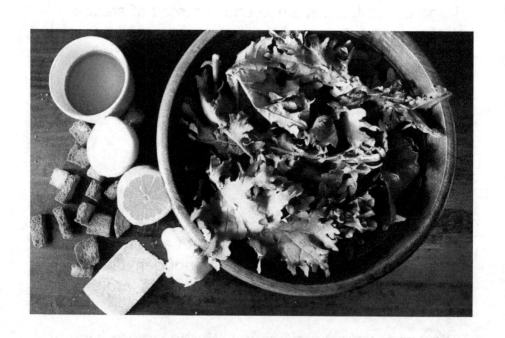

Venison Tenderloin

Preparation time: 20 minutes

Cooking time: 75 minutes

Servings: 6

Ingredients:

4 pounds venison tenderloin

2 sprigs fresh thyme

2 sprigs fresh rosemary

2 cloves garlic, crushed 2

2 bay leaves

1 medium onion, chopped

1 cup red wine

½ cup apple cider vinegar

Directions:

1.Add red wine cider vinegar, garlic, bay leaves, thyme, rosemary & onion in a cup & blend them.

2.Move it to the large jar, & place in the bag the venison tenderloin.

3.Close it tightly, and make it airtight.

4.Then place the meat in a refrigerator for marination for at least 13 hours, turn it 2 or 3 times.

5.Preheated the oven to 325ºF (165 ºC).

6.Take Off meat away from the marinade & put it in a roasting rack.

7.Roast it for two to two and a half hours in the oven.

8.The Internal roasting temperature would be a minimum of 150 ºF

9.Let the roast rest for 10 to 15 minutes before cutting.

10Heat the sauce over low heat in a pan as the side roasts.

11.Boil till there is a 1/3 drop in the oil. Serve & Enjoy

Seared venison with plum ginger sauce and vermicelli sauce

Preparation time: 10 minutes

Cooking time: 15 minutes

Servings: 2

Ingredients:

Vermicelli salad

carrot grated

1red capsicum sliced

100snow peas sliced

1100 g vermicelli noodles

2 tbsp Thai basil leaves chopped Venison and plum sauce

¼ cup red wine

1 clove garlic minced 1

 tablespoon soy sauce

1 teaspoon ginger finely grated

2 tablespoons plum jam

300 g venison medallions Dressing

½ teaspoon sesame oil

1 tablespoon olive oil

1 tablespoon soy sauce

1 teaspoon plum jam

To serve

2 tablespoon Thai basil leaves chopped 1

 tablespoon sesame seeds

Directions:

1.Bring to the boil a full pot.

2.Use a Proof heat Bowl, place the vermicelli noodles in the bowl and pour over the boiling water to cover them.

3.Threads are detached by stirring, covering with a plate, and leaving until smooth, around 4 minutes. 4

4.Threads are shortened by cutting the threads from different places using kitchen scissors. Apply oil in a small amount to avoid Sticking.

5.Use paper towels, Dry the venison, and season it with salt. Heat the saucepan to medium temperature. Toast sesame seeds until crispy and fragrant for 1 to 2 minutes.

6.Add a drizzle of oil and raise the heat. Once cooked, grill the venison for 2 to 3 minutes on both sides. Cover the venison with foil.

7.Return the pan to low heat for the plum sauce and apply a small amount of oil. Fry the ginger and garlic for 30 seconds, stir-fry the red wine, and boil until halved. Now add plum jelly, fresh plums, and soy sauce and boil until slightly thickened, and stir for around 1 minute.

8.Use black pepper for seasoning. If the sauce gets too thick and jam-like, give a splash of water to thin it out to a decent pouring consistency. Stir in the sleeping venison juices.

9.Mix all of the ingredients in a big dish. Add all the salad ingredients leftover, the noodles, and toss to coat. Season with salt and pepper.

10.Divide the vermicelli salad between the plates to serve. Cover with venison and drizzle all over the sauce with plum. Sprinkle the Thai basil and sesame seeds.

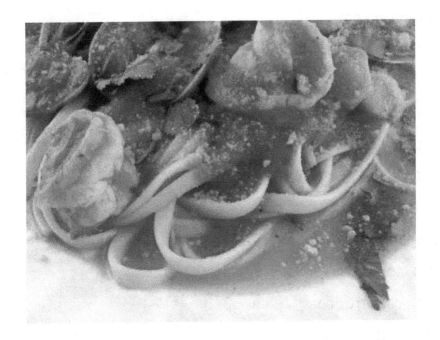

Venison Stir-Fry

Preparation time: 20 minutes

Cooking time: 5 minutes

Servings: 4

Ingredients:

Marinade

1/2 teaspoon salt

2 tablespoons Shaoxing wine or dry sherry

3 tablespoons soy sauce

1 tablespoon potato starch stir fry

1 1/2 cups peanut or other cooking oil

1 pound venison, trimmed of fat

1 to 4 fresh red chiles

1 red or yellow bell pepper, sliced

3 garlic cloves, slivered

1 bunch cilantro, roughly chopped

1 tablespoon soy sauce

2 teaspoons sesame oil

Directions:

1.Cut the venison into small slivers between 1/4 inch or less and 1 to 3 inches in length from anywhere.

2.Mix and set aside with the marinade as you cut out all the remaining ingredients.

3.Heat a big heavy pot with the peanut oil until it reaches 275 °F to 290°F.

4.Apply about 1/3 of venison to hot oil and use a chopstick or   a butter knife to separate the meat slices. Let them sizzle for 30 - 60 seconds.

5.Set aside and cook one-third at a time for the remaining venison.

6.Pour all but only three tablespoons of the oil out of it.

7.Keep the remaining oil hot. Add up the chiles and the bell peppers. Stir-fry for 90 seconds when it starts to burn, add garlic, and cook for an extra 30 seconds.

8.Add the venison and fry for 90 seconds and stir.

9.Add the coriander and soy sauce and fry for the remaining 30 seconds before the coriander wilts. Turn the heat off, then whisk in the sesame oil.

10.Serve with steamed rice at once.

Lamb, apricot & shallot tagine

Preparation time: 30 minutes

Cooking time: 7 hrs 30 minutes

Servings: 5-6

Ingredients:

1 tbsp clear honey

1 tbsp ras el hanout

One large leg of lamb, bone-in (about 2kg)

150ml hot chicken stock

2 preserved lemons

400g small apricot, halved and stoned

600g shallot, halved if particularly large

85g whole skinless almond couscous and natural yogurt, to serve little pack coriander leaves picked

For the marinade

1 tbsp ground cumin

2 tbsp clear honey

1 tsp coriander seed

2 tsp ground cinnamon

2 tsp ground ginger

4 tbsp olive oil

4 garlic cloves, crushed pinch of saffron strands

Directions:

1.Cut the lamb's leg all over and put it in a large bag of food. Using the pestle and mortar, shatter the marinade ingredients simultaneously. Brush over the entire lamb with black pepper. Overnight, or up to 24 hours, to marinate.

2.Place the lamb in a large roasting tin, removing any residual marinade from the top. Use foil to protect the container, and close the foil from the ends. Cook for 6-7 hours, basting until the beef is extremely tender.

3.Drop the oven roasting tin and raise the oven to 200ºC /180ºC. Pour into a measuring jug the juices from the lamb, slightly cool it, and remove the fat off.

4.Place the shallots with the lamb in the tin and toss in some of the juices to coat them. Roast the apricots and almonds for 15 mins, and then add them.

5.Whisk the lemon, honey, ras el hanout, and stock in the cooking juices, then pour on the lamb and then roast again for 20 mins.

6.Leave it for 10 minutes, then scatter and eat with couscous and yogurt over the herbs.

Flank Steak, Broccoli and Green Bean Stir-Fry

Preparation time: 15minutes

Cooking time: 12minutes

Servings:

Ingredients:

3 cups cooked brown rice

2 tablespoons vegetable oil

2 tablespoons rice vinegar

1¼ pound lean beef flank steak

1 cup beef broth

1 tablespoon cornstarch

1 head broccoli, cut into florets (about 6 cups)

1 cup shredded carrot

½ teaspoon red pepper flakes

½ teaspoon Chinese five-spice powder

½ pound thin green beans, trimmed

½ large onion, sliced

½ cup sliced almonds

¼ teaspoon salt

¼ cup reduced-sodium soy sauce

Directions:

1.Combine the soy sauce, broth, 5-spice powder, vinegar, cornstarch, & the red chili flakes in a cup and place it aside.

2.Take a non-stick fry pan, add 1 tbsp of oil to it, and heat it. Pepper the salted stir-fry flank steak & for 4 minutes. Remove to a tray.

3.Add the remaining one tbsp. Of oil in it, and then add broccoli, cabbage, green beans, & carrot. Stir-cook for 9 minutes or till it becomes soft & crisp.

4.Add ¼ cup of water at the last two minutes of cooking time.

5.Now add a mixture of soya sauce& broth in it and then boil & simmer it for 2 minutes, until well dense. Stir in some stored juices & beef & heat up.

6.Decorate with the almonds & serve with the cooked brown rice instantly.

Persian Roast Lamb

Preparation time: 20 minutes

Cooking time: 150 minutes

Servings: 8

Ingredients:

1 large onion sliced or chopped

1 tbsp EV olive oil

1 tbsp ground cumin

1 tsp ground black pepper

1 tsp turmeric

1 leg or shoulder of lamb

Two strips of fresh rosemary 2 Tbsp honey

Tbsp liquid saffron

250 ml of vegetable stock

4 tbsp pomegranate molasses

5. cloves garlic finely chopped or crushed One lemon juice

Directions:

1.Preheat micro to 180 deg C.

2.Make slashes.

3.Mix ingredients & rub them over the lamb.

4.Line sliced onions with a preferred dish.

5.Pour the stock.

6.Remember to Pour on onions.

7.Cover using foil & roast for 60 minutes.

8.Have the lamb wrapped in aluminum foil with a wonderful sauce.

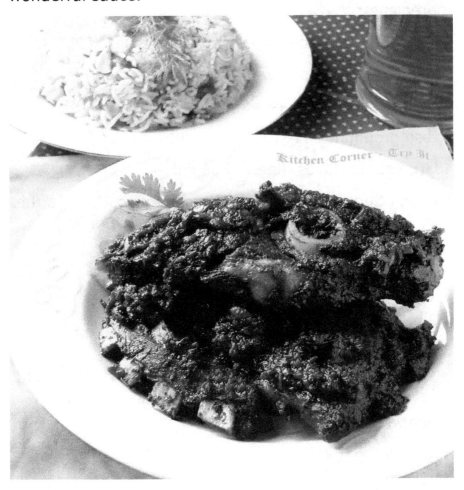

Stir-fried garlic chili beef and ong Choi

Preparation time: 8 minutes

Cooking time: 15 minutes

Servings: 2

Ingredients:

200g beef fillet, sliced into even-sized thin strips

Few pinches Chinese five-spice

Light soy sauce to season

1 tbsp groundnut oil

4 large garlic cloves, finely chopped

150 ong Choi, washed, leaves and stems cut across the stem in equal 10cm lengths (or use spinach or watercress)

1 medium red chili, de-seeded and finely chopped
Toasted sesame oil, to season

Directions:

1.Season the beef with soy sauce.

2.Toss well.

3.Heat a saucepan.

4.Add oil & garlic.

5.Fry 30 sec.

6.Add beef & stir.

7.Apply one Choi & chili.

8.Season with light soy sauce, sea salt, & sesame oil splashes for serving.

9.Serve immediately & enjoy.

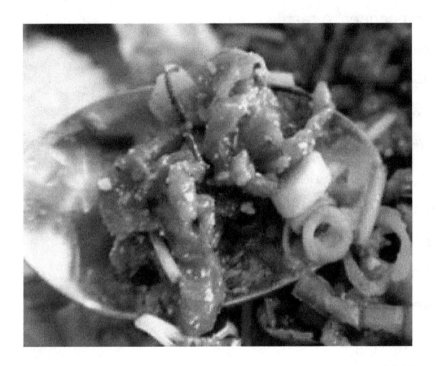

Asian Broccoli and Ginger Salad

Preparation time: 10minutes

Cooking time: 10 minutes

Servings: 4

Ingredients:

Salt and pepper to taste

3 tablespoons low sodium soy sauce

3 tablespoons balsamic vinegar

2 cloves garlic minced

2 teaspoons brown sugar

2 cups sugar snap peas

1/4 cup almonds

1 red pepper julienne cut

1 (12 ounces) bag broccoli coleslaw

1 tablespoon fresh ginger

1 1/2 teaspoons sesame oil

Directions:

1.Mix soy sauce, garlic, sesame oil, vinegar, brown sugar, & ginger.

2.Put it aside for a while.

3.Steam sugar snaps for roughly 3-4 min.

4.For stopping the cooking process, immerse it in an ice bath.

5.Drain well.

6.Mix peas, almonds, broccoli coleslaw, red pepper & sesame ginger.

7.Dressing in a big dish.

8.Add salt to taste & black pepper powder.

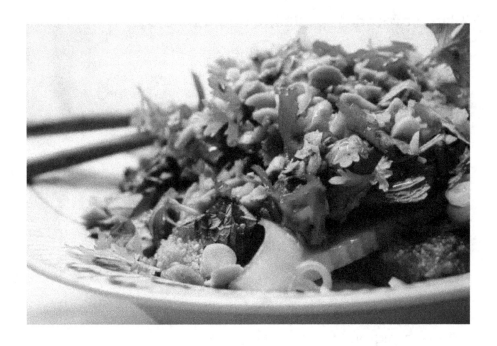

Avocado and three-bean salad

Preparation time: 15minutes

Cooking time: 15 minutes

Servings: 8

Ingredients:

Salt and pepper to taste juice of 2 limes

2 large avocados, peeled, pitted, and diced

2 cloves garlic, mashed or finely diced

12 grape or cherry tomatoes, halved

1/3 cup olive oil

1 large orange or red bell pepper, diced

1 bunch cilantro, chopped

15 oz kernel corn

15 oz red kidney beans

15 oz garbanzo beans 15 oz black beans

Directions:

1.Take a big bowl.

2.Combine all ingredients.

3.Refrigerate for 60 minutes before serving.

4.Tossed it with lime.

5.Serve & enjoy.

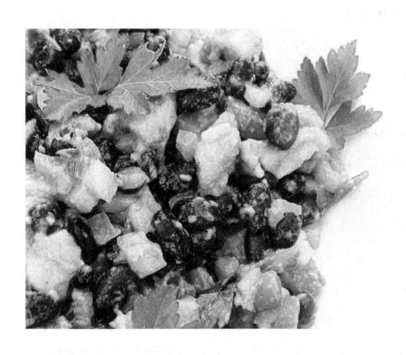

Baked Adzuki Beans with Aubergine & Tomatoes

Preparation time: 8 minutes

Cooking time: 90 minutes

Servings: 6

Ingredients:

1 bouquet garni (thyme, parsley, and bay leaf)

1 cup chicken stock (or one bouillon cube dissolved in 1 cup water)

1 cup dried adzuki beans

One onion, finely chopped

1/2 cup fresh grated parmesan cheese

1/2 teaspoon ground allspice

1/4 teaspoon red pepper flakes

2 cloves garlic, minced

2 sliced eggplants

1/2 cups canned chopped tomatoes Four tablespoons fresh basil, shredded

6 tablespoons olive oil

kosher salt or sea salt

Salt and pepper, to taste

Directions:

1.Add garlic & boil water.

2.Reduce heat & simmer before beans become soft for 50 minutes.

3.Preheat microwave to 375°.

4.Heat olive oil in a frying pan on moderate heat.

5.Move to bake dish.

6.Heat leftover olive oil pan & sauté onion before it begins to soften.

7.Add garlic & sauté for one min.

8.Add tomatoes, red pepper flakes, salt, allspice, & black pepper.

9.Blend well.

10Sprinkle with cheese & bake for 20 min.

11.Serve & enjoy.

Roasted Sorghum

Preparation Time: 10 minutes

Cooking Time: 15 minutes

Servings: 4

Ingredients:

1 tbsp. avocado oil

½ cup sorghum, cooked

1 carrot, diced

1 tbsp. dried parsley

½ tsp. dried oregano

2 tbsp. cream cheese

Directions:

1.Heat avocado oil and add the carrot.

2.Roast it for 5 minutes.

3.Then add cooked sorghum, parsley, oregano, and cream cheese.

4.Roast the meal for 10 minutes on low heat. Stir it from time to time to avoid burning.

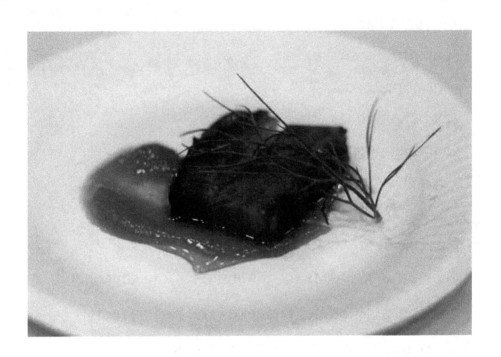

Sorghum Stew

Preparation Time: 10 minutes

Cooking Time: 25 minutes

Servings: 5

Ingredients:

1 cup sorghum

½ cup ground sausages

½ cup tomatoes

1 jalapeno pepper, chopped

½ cup bell pepper, chopped

4 cups chicken stock

Directions:

1.Roast the sausages for 5 minutes in the saucepan.

2.Then add tomatoes, jalapeno, and bell pepper.

3.Cook the ingredients for 10 minutes.

4.After this, add sorghum and chicken stock and boil the stew for 10 minutes more.

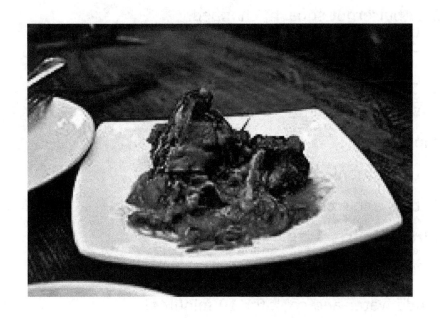

Sorghum Salad

Preparation Time: 10 minutes

Cooking Time: 10 minutes

Servings: 3

Ingredients:

3 oz butternut squash, chopped

¼ cup sorghum

¼ cup fresh cilantro, chopped

1 tsp. ground cumin

cups water

2 tbsp. organic canola oil

2 tbsp. apple cider vinegar

Directions:

1.Put sorghum and butternut squash in the saucepan.

2.Add water and cook for 10 minutes.

3.Then cool the ingredients and transfer in the salad bowl.

4.Add cilantro, ground cumin, organic canola oil, and apple cider vinegar.

5.Stir the meal well.

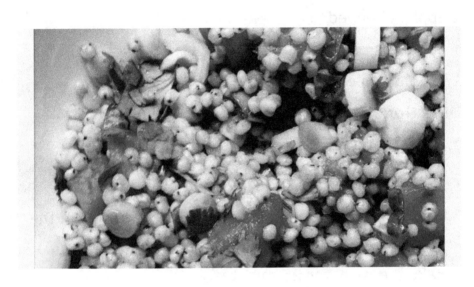

Sorghum Bake

Preparation Time: 10 minutes

Cooking Time: 25 minutes

Servings: 4

Ingredients:

½ cup sorghum

1 apple, chopped

1 oz raisins

1.5cup of water

Directions:

1.Put sorghum in the pan. Flatten it.

2.Then top it with raisins, apple, and water.

3.Cover the meal with baking paper and transfer in the preheated to 375F oven.

4.Bake the meal for 25 minutes.

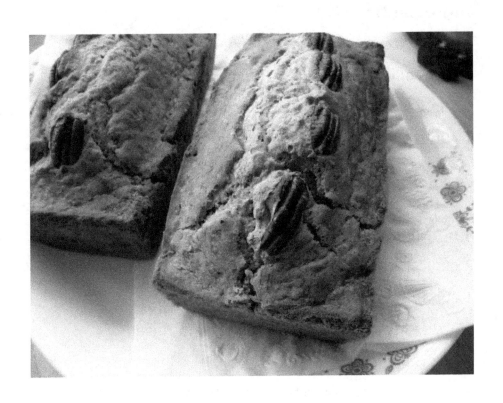

Lamb and Chickpeas Stew

Preparation Time: 10 minutes

Cooking Time: 1 hour and 20 minutes

Servings: 6

Ingredients:

1 and ½ lb. lamb shoulder, cubed

3 tbsp. olive oil

1 cup yellow onion, chopped

1 cup carrots, cubed

1 cup celery, chopped

3 garlic cloves, minced

4 rosemary springs, chopped

2 cups chicken stock

1 cup tomato puree

15 oz. canned chickpeas, drained and rinsed

10 oz. baby spinach

2 tbsp. black olives, pitted and sliced

A pinch of salt and black pepper

Directions:

1.Heat a pot with the oil over medium-high heat, add the meat, salt and pepper and brown for 5 minutes.

2.Add carrots, celery, onion and garlic, stir and sauté for 5 minutes more.

3.Add the rosemary, stock, chickpeas and the other ingredients except the spinach and olives, stir and cook for 1 hour.

4.Add the rest of the ingredients, cook the stew over medium heat for 10 minutes more, divide into bowls and serve.

Chorizo and Lentils Stew

Preparation Time: 10 minutes

Cooking Time: 35 minutes

Servings: 4

Ingredients:

4 cups water

1 cup carrots, sliced

1 yellow onion, chopped

1 tbsp. extra-virgin olive oil

¾ cup celery, chopped

1 and ½ tsp. garlic, minced

1 and ½ lb. gold potatoes, roughly chopped

7 oz. chorizo, cut in half lengthwise and thinly sliced

1 and ½ cup lentils

½ tsp. smoked paprika

½ tsp. oregano

Salt and black pepper to taste

14 oz. canned tomatoes, chopped

½ cup cilantro, chopped

Directions:

1.Heat a saucepan with oil over medium high heat, add onion, garlic, celery and carrots, stir and cook for 4 minutes.

2.Add the chorizo, stir and cook for 1 minute more.

3.Add the rest of the ingredients except the cilantro, stir, bring to a boil, reduce heat to medium-low and simmer for 25 minutes.

4.Divide the stew into bowls and serve with the cilantro sprinkled on top. Enjoy!

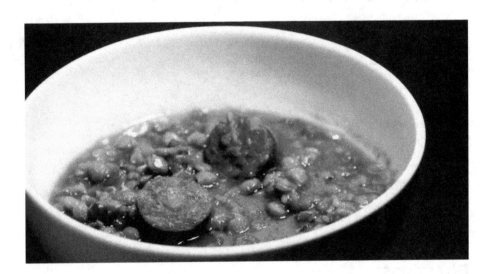

Lamb and Potato Stew

Preparation Time: 10 minutes

Cooking Time: 2 hours

Servings: 4

Ingredients:

2 and ½ lb. lamb shoulder, boneless and cut in small pieces

Salt and black pepper to taste

1 yellow onion, chopped

3 tbsp. extra virgin olive oil

3 tomatoes, grated

and ½ cups chicken stock

½ cup dry white wine

1 bay leaf and ½ lb. gold potatoes, cut into medium cubes

¾ cup green olives

Directions:

1.Heat a saucepan with the oil over medium high heat, add the lamb, brown for 10 minutes, transfer to a platter and keep warm for now.

2.Heat the pan again, add onion, stir and cook for 4 minutes.

3.Add tomatoes, stir, reduce heat to low and cook for 15 minutes.

4.Return lamb meat to pan, add wine and the rest of the ingredients except the potatoes and olives, stir, increase heat to medium high, bring to a boil, reduce heat again, cover pan and simmer for 30 minutes.

5.Add potatoes and olives, stir, cook for 1 more hour., divide into bowls and serve.

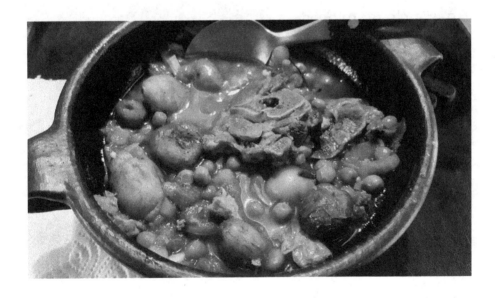

Meatball and Pasta Soup

Preparation Time: 10 minutes

Cooking Time: 40 minutes

Servings: 4

Ingredients:

12 oz. pork meat, ground

12 oz. veal, ground

Salt and black pepper to taste

1 garlic clove, minced

garlic cloves, sliced

2 tsp. thyme, chopped

1 egg, whisked

oz. Manchego, grated

2 tbsp. extra virgin olive oil

1/3 cup panko

4 cups chicken stock

A pinch of saffron

15 oz. canned tomatoes, crushed

1 tbsp. parsley, chopped

8 oz. pasta

Directions:

1.In a bowl, mix veal with pork, 1 garlic clove, 1 tsp. thyme,¼ tsp. paprika, salt, pepper to taste, egg, manchego, panko, stir very well and shape medium meatballs out of this mix.

2.Heat a pan with 1 ½ tbsp. oil over medium high heat, add half of the meatballs, cook for 2 minutes on each side, transfer to paper towels, drain grease and put on a plate.

3.Repeat this with the rest of the meatballs.

4.Heat a saucepan with the rest of the oil, add sliced garlic, stir and cook for 1 minute.

5.Add the remaining ingredients and the meatballs, stir, reduce heat to medium low, cook for 25 minutes and season with salt and pepper.

6.Cook pasta according to instructions, drain, put in a bowl and mix with ½ cup soup.

7.Divide pasta into soup bowls, add soup and meatballs on top, sprinkle parsley all over and serve.

Peas Soup

Preparation Time: 10 minutes

Cooking Time: 10 minutes

Servings: 4

Ingredients:

1 tsp. shallot, chopped

1 tbsp. butter

quart chicken stock 2 eggs

3 tbsp. lemon juice 2 cups peas

2 tbsp. parmesan, grated

Salt and black pepper to taste

Directions:

1.Heat a saucepan with the butter over medium high heat, add shallot, stir and cook for 2 minutes.

2.Add stock, lemon juice, some salt and pepper and the whisked eggs .

3.Add more salt and pepper to taste, peas and parmesan cheese, stir, cook for 3 minutes, divide into bowls and serve.

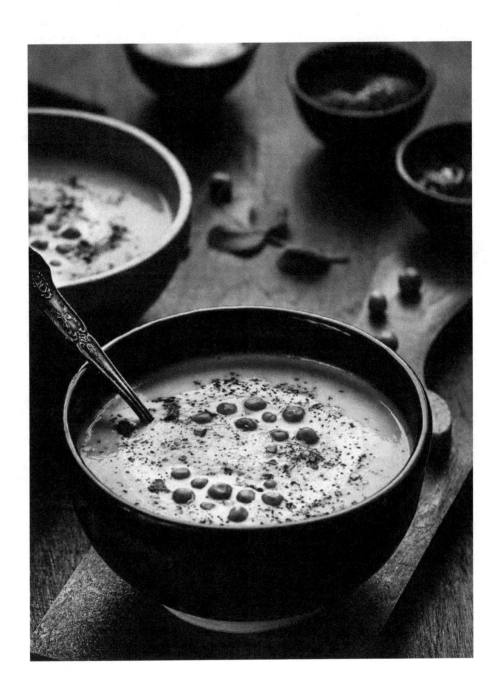

Minty Lamb Stew

Preparation Time: 10 minutes

Cooking Time: 1 hour and 45 minutes

Servings: 4

Ingredients:

1 cups orange juice

½ cup mint tea

Salt and black pepper to taste

2 lb. lamb shoulder chops

1 tbsp. mustard, dry

3 tbsp. canola oil

1 tbsp. ras el hanout

1 carrot, chopped

1 yellow onion, chopped

1 celery rib, chopped

1 tbsp. ginger, grated

28 oz. canned tomatoes, crushed

1 tbsp. garlic, mincedstar anise

1 cup apricots, dried and cut in halves

1 cinnamon stick

½ cup mint, chopped

15 oz. canned chickpeas, drained 6 tbsp. yogurt

Directions:

1.Put orange juice in a saucepan, bring to a boil over medium heat, take off heat, add tea leaves, cover and leave aside for 3 minutes, strain this and leave aside.

2.Heat a saucepan with 2 tbsp. oil over medium high heat, add lamb chops seasoned with salt, pepper, mustard and rasel hanout, toss, brown for 3 minutes on each side and transfer to a plate.

3.Add remaining oil to the saucepan, heat over medium heat, add ginger, onion, carrot, garlic and celery, stir and cook for 5 minutes.

4.Add orange juice, star anise, tomatoes, cinnamon stick, lamb, apricots, stir and cook for 1 hour and 30 minutes.

5.Transfer lamb chops to a cutting board, discard bones and chop.

6.Bring sauce from the pan to a boil, add chickpeas and mint, stir and cook for 10 minutes.

7.Discard cinnamon and star anise, divide into bowls and serve with yogurt on top.

Spinach and Orzo Soup

Preparation Time: 10 minutes

Cooking Time: 10 minutes

Servings: 4

Ingredients:

½ cup orzo

6 cups chicken soup and ½ cups parmesan, grated

Salt and black pepper to taste

1 and ½ tsp. oregano, dried

¼ cup yellow onion, finely chopped

3 cups baby spinach

1 tbsp. lemon juice

½ cup peas, frozen

Directions:

1.Heat a saucepan with the stock over high heat, add oregano, orzo, onion, salt and pepper, stir, bring to a boil, cover and cook for 10 minutes.

2.Take soup off the heat, add salt and pepper to taste and the rest of the ingredients , stir well and divide into soup bowls. Serve right away.

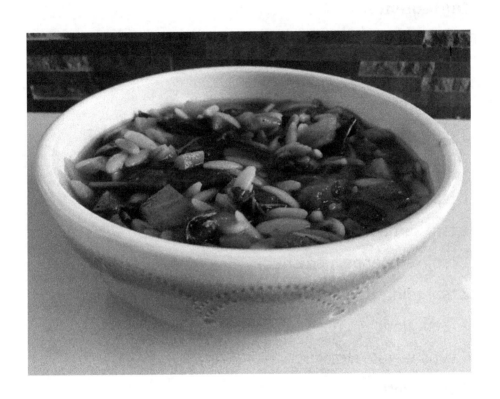

Minty Lentil and Spinach Soup

Preparation Time: 10 minutes

Cooking Time: 30 minutes

Servings: 6

Ingredients:

2 tbsp. olive oil

1 yellow onion, chopped

A pinch of salt and black pepper

2 garlic cloves, minced

1 tsp. coriander, ground

1 tsp. cumin, ground

1 tsp. sumac

1 tsp. red pepper, crushed

2 tsp. mint, dried

1 tbsp. flour

6 cups veggie stock

3 cups water

12 oz. spinach, torn

1 and ½ cups brown lentils, rinsed

2 cups parsley, chopped

Juice of 1 lime

Directions:

1.Heat a pot with the oil over medium heat, add the onions, stir and sauté for 5 minutes.

2.Add garlic, salt, pepper, coriander, cumin, sumac, red pepper, mint and flour, stir and cook for another minute.

3.Add the stock, water and the other ingredients except the parsley and lime juice, stir, bring to a simmer and cook for 20 minutes.

4.Add the parsley and lime juice, cook the soup for 5 minutes more, ladle into bowls and serve.

Chicken and Apricots Stew

Preparation Time: 10 minutes

Cooking Time: 2 hours and 10 minutes

Servings: 4

Ingredients:

3 garlic cloves, minced

1 tbsp. parsley, chopped 20 saffron threads

3 tbsp. cilantro, chopped

Salt and black pepper to taste

1 tsp. ginger, ground

tbsp. olive oil

red onions, thinly sliced

4 chicken drumsticks

5 oz. apricots, dried 2 tbsp. butter

¼ cup honey

2/3 cup walnuts, chopped

½ cinnamon stick

Directions:

1.Heat a pan over medium high heat, add saffron threads, toast them for 2 minutes, transfer to a bowl, cool down and crush.

2.Add the chicken pieces, 1 tbsp. cilantro, parsley, garlic, ginger, salt, pepper, oil and 2 tbsp. water, toss well and keep in the fridge for 30 minutes.

3.Arrange onion on the bottom of a saucepan.

4.Add chicken and marinade, add 1 tbsp. butter, place on stove over medium high heat and cook for 15 minutes.

5.Add ¼ cup water, stir, cover pan, reduce heat to medium- low and simmer for 45 minutes.

6.Heat a pan over medium heat, add 2 tbsp. honey, cinnamon stick, apricots and ¾ cup water, stir, bring to a boil, reduce to low and simmer for 15 minutes.

7.Take off heat, discard cinnamon and leave to cool down.

8.Heat a pan with remaining butter over medium heat, add remaining honey and walnuts, stir, cook for 5 minutes and transfer to a plate.

9.Add chicken to apricot sauce, also season with salt, pepper and the rest of the cilantro stir, cook for 10 minutes and serve on top of walnuts.

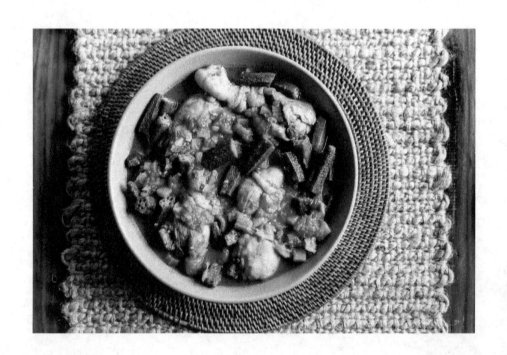